Eat Better

By Bryan Frawley

A guide that will make you feel so much better

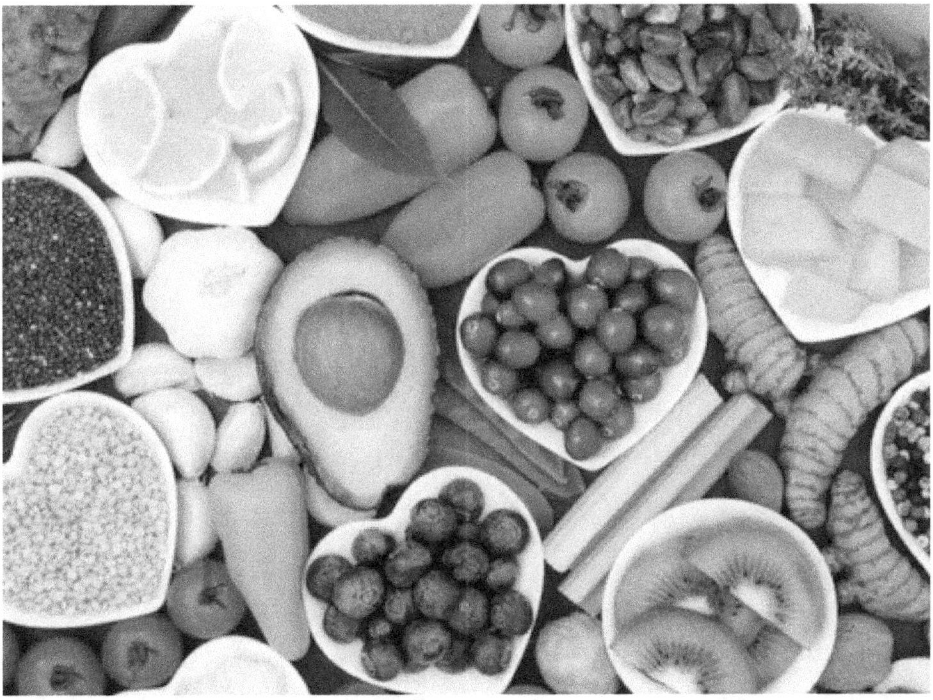

Table of contents

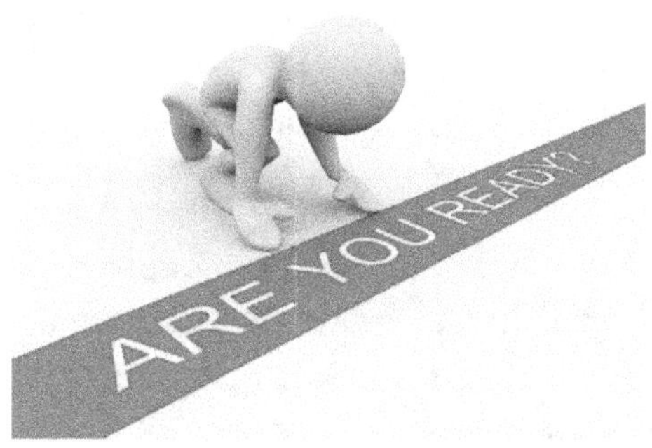

This book needs to start with a slight rant. We've been taught how to eat by a generation who was told what to do by the news. There is also a status quo that comes with this generation. They might say, oh it's ok live a little (which they don't mean a little, more like often), or your belly pudge is fine. Why can't we be better than this? We have the knowledge and ability to eat better yet we don't. It's because we were taught this way and we have all heard fad diets don't work. What I present isn't a fad diet, I am presenting a better plan to live by so you can grow old with much less chances of getting diseases.

 The same generation doesn't understand portions, has also been the generation with the most heart related issues. We need to learn from them and be better. This isn't a hate mantra against certain generations. My goal is to give you the tools to change your thinking. Poor eating will lead to poor health later in life and even now as well.

The plan I have studied had allowed me to lose weight, yes. But what I really like about the plan is, I feel better, I sleep better, my energy is better, and I do better in the sack. When I used to eat poorly I can remember how tired I was, and when I tried to workout, that didn't go as well either. Changing what I ate was the difference maker.

There are plenty out there who say, I can outwork a bad diet and stay in shape. That's cool, I was 22 once before too. Now in my 30's, I learned that isn't possible anymore, your body changes. Your body needs certain nutrients that you just can't get from a medium pizza and a 6-pack. That was my busy life while active duty in the Marines too, big difference.

If you are in your 30's or 40's and have a ton of pains, headaches, and are extremely tired. You need to know this isn't normal. You can fix this by adjusting your diet. Most will just write this off and say, oh I must be getting old. As someone in their mid-30's I was having those pains and just thought maybe it was my body worn out from my time in the Marines. Even with how hard I pushed my body then, it shouldn't reflect now.

Full disclaimer before reading too far. I am a huge fan of craft beer and I consume in moderation I haven't removed alcohol from my diet and with that I still am losing weight. The key is moderation and balance. I tend to keep my limit to two in one night. When I do go out if I have more than one or two, I mix in a glass of water here and there. I mention this as I preach moderation, but mostly to say you don't need to cut this out of your life.

This isn't a vegetarian only diet but does include a lot of vegetables. You can't get these vitamins and nutrients from a multi-vitamin or a pill. The multivitamin shelves are mostly filled with synthetic lab made nutrients, as you can imagine, this isn't what your body needs.

Another key here is, adjusting your diet and lifestyle as the long-term fix, not short term. As mentioned, this isn't a fad diet to try and see what happens. This will be a lifestyle change and I will explain some science on a simple level of why.

You can save your money with all of the pills out there, they are polluting your body. Most of the vitamins in vitamin supplements don't even absorb into your body anyhow. Think about it, those vitamins are made in a lab!

Here is the best part. Yes, you will lose weight. Yes you will look better. That is just the outside benefits. You will feel better, have more energy, be mentally stronger, and have a better outlook on relationships, life and opportunities.

I will break down some different categories to look at improving that all work together. Each category is separate but connected.

Water

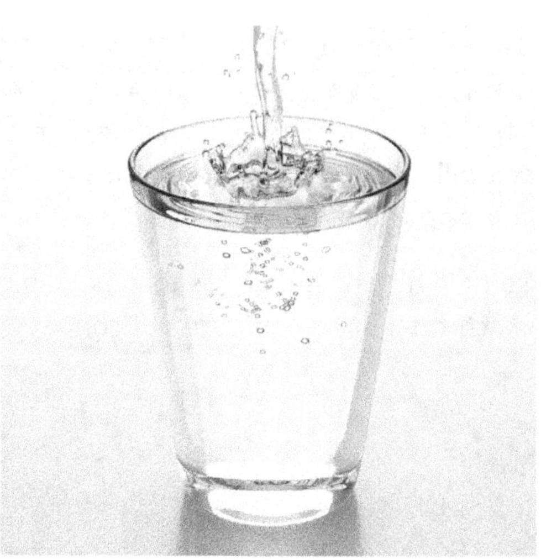

To me water is the most important part of being healthy, and my number one priority. I am sure you have heard, you can go days and weeks without food, but only two days without water. In those two days you would have already created some damage to your body. Later I will talk about acid VS alkalinity, water plays a major role in your overall balance.

Water is basically how our entire body functions. And without water, your body doesn't function.

Water is a part of your digestion. In fact sometimes when you think you are hungry it is usually just be your body's way of asking for water. The hungry signal your brain is sent from the stomach can't tell if it is hunger or thirst.

Start your day off with a glass of water. Your body loses water when you sleep, before you put something acidic in your body (that first sip of coffee), you want to have water in your system. Your body loses a lot of water in your sleep when breathing, and you lose it through your sweat glands. Replacing what was drained is vital.

Your saliva is made of water, which contains enzymes to help break down food. Fun fact, broccoli and your saliva enzymes mixed together adds a chemical combination for an added benefit of broccoli (more on that in the food section).

Water regulates your body temperature. One way to prevent the flu or at least prep your body to fight hard is to just be hydrated. Water helps lubricate and cushion joints, and your spinal cord.

You excrete toxins and waste because of water, with sweat, urination and helping bowel movements. Drinking enough water helps kidney's be more efficient and prevents kidney stones.

Without water and enough of it, your body can achieve maximum physical performance. Strength, power and endurance are all effected by your level of hydration. In the same subject of exercise, water carries oxygen in your blood stream improving your circulation.

Feeling down? Slam a glass of water, moodiness can come from lack of hydration.

How much should you drink? National Academies of Sciences say about 125 ounces each day for men and 91 ounces for women.

Water consumption doesn't come from just drinking a glass. Around 10-20% of your daily water intake will come from food. Include in your diet lots of fruits and bright colored vegetables including raw vegetables.

Water shouldn't just come from any source. Do research on the source of your water. Most bottled water is actually crap and doesn't even have minerals you need. Spring water bottles are typically the best, but is not the best source, only go for this when you are need.

A national survey shows around 75% of the country is dehydrated. This is a shocking statistic and you should consider making sure you are not part of this number!

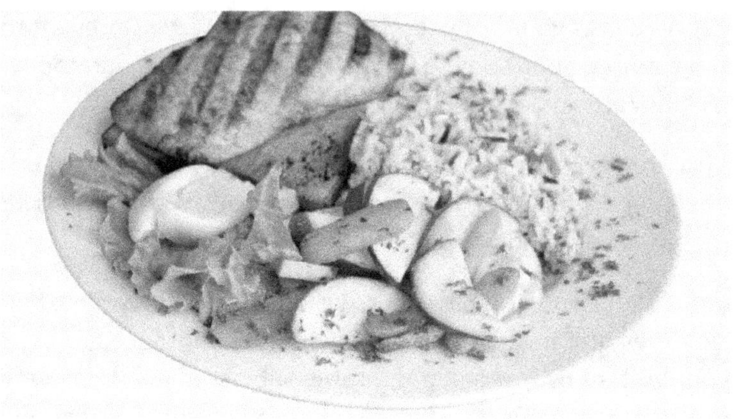

There can't be enough to say about watch what you are eating. Watching how much you eat per meal is just as key. For instance, I am not going to shame you for eating a cheeseburger. Just watch how often you do so.

Quite honestly, the word track of "oh I don't eat what my food eats" or "I like to taste my food" is complete crap. Lots of foods I will suggest in the writing and at the end of this book in a neat list for you, are tasty. The best part is, you don't feel like you need a doctor and/or a nap after you are done with a meal.

In my past I used to eat whatever and get seconds, this included burgers, fast food, and polishing off a few slices of pizza. The problem is, we did this often and I never balanced it all out. My biggest game changer that made me more aware and made me set out to learn more is making one change.

That change was removing breakfast frozen burritos every morning (for convenience) and replacing with oatmeal. This change dropped 5 pounds for me in about a month. And I didn't change anything else in my diet or exercise. The pure amount of food didn't change much at all, in fact they weighed about the same and calories weren't that far off. The difference was the nutrients, way less saturated fats, and now full of whole grains.

What I learned is, eating something often that is sweet and higher in fats causes more than I knew. Where my old way of thinking was, if I work off these many calories I will be good, right? Wrong! I had this mentality in the Marines. I would eat absolutely horrible foods and I was still in good shape. Well as you can imagine, Marines are super active. Once I got out of the Marines I gained weight right away, and would fluctuate for years as well.

Eating a 400 calorie donut once in awhile isn't going to hurt you. But eating too much sugar often can raise blood pressure, trigger inflammation and raise triglycerides. These are all major risks of heart diseases. Speaking of donuts, aside form the sugar overload there are also synthetic flavors, additives, preservatives and trans fats. Remember in the intro chapter talking about "growing pains" in your 30's? This is from too much sugar and other crap causing inflammation.

Next I started making other changes with adding more leafy greens with tons of vegetables. Que, the I don't want to eat what my food eats, don't worry we will cover meat later. I removed chips and other junk from my diet, there goes another 5 pounds! I really need to tell you, finishing a whole vegetable meal feels great walking away from the table. Now flip the script, walking away from the table from a ½ pound burger with cheese and bacon, then a large side of fries, you know you walk away from that table hating yourself. Don't tell me you don't.

What I concentrate on is fruits for snacking instead, grapes, apples, bananas, and a lot of melons like cantaloupe, watermelon especially. Also for snacks I include seeds like sprouted pumpkin seeds I got from Costco, and cashews (non-acid forming). These also make great snacks and will generally fill you up when eating proper portions.

Additionally, nuts and seeds are high in fiber, protein and heart-healthy fats. The contain anti-inflammatory and antioxidant properties. Other nuts and seeds to consider, sunflower seeds, chia seeds, flaxseeds and help seeds. Did you know, for vitamins to be digested and absorbed for your body to benefit, you need healthy fats.

For breakfast I typically have oatmeal still, the brand is Kodiak cakes, it's a heartier whole grains oatmeal, but it does have its share of sugar. So instead every couple of days I substitute with steel cut oats. I will also have berries with breakfast as well which are all on the alkaline side (as opposed to acidic), including raspberries, strawberries, blueberries, and cranberries.

During the day I try to drink green tea over extra coffee. Green tea is full of antioxidants and polyphenolic compounds which have strong anti-inflammatory effects. I will say it again, moderation. I still drink coffee first, and sometimes in the afternoon. However I try to balance that with a water, and choose green tea when possible.

Lunch will typically be a salad full of greens especially spinach. In the salad will be peppers, cucumbers, raw broccoli, raw cauliflower and no dressing. The dressing can be added just watch what you do add. I will sometime have a cut up chicken breast on the salad but not always.

Dinner, I will usually play the substitution game with my family. For instance, we used to use our air fryer for fries (not heavily), but now we cut up potatoes and air fry them, these won't have preservatives or added sugars. While the family does that, I took it a step further and cut up a sweet potato, I will get one of my kids to like those one day! Sweat potatoes are one of the most nutrient dense foods you can eat as well!

As we look through the stores we try to find good substitutes for foods that are still fun to eat. For instance, we found a cauliflower pizza that is full of veggies. Instead of a flour-based dough, it is cauliflower, it's still delicious and is more nutritious. If you can make just a few small changes at the store, you will benefit much more than you think.

The more you look at labels the better as well. I will go over processed foods in a different chapter. But knowing which foods are included in your choices at the store are going to help you a lot. An entire book could be written on processed foods and label reading, so take a good look and build on that knowledge after reading this book.

If you know you are going out to dinner try researching the menu early for healthy choices. Often once the menu is in front of you, you might feel rushed if the rest of the table is ready to order. If you already did your research to know what the healthiest option could be, you will be armed with a better plan.

If your yard or property permits it (harder in subdivisions), try growing a garden. Having your own source of fresh veggies and fruits is awesome. A little work will help you feel good too. Chances are, most readers are in office jobs. Switching up your night and weekend routine with some outside work will be good for you.

Think of healthier eating as a process. The more you change what you eat, the more you will crave those foods instead.

My favorite healthy food objection is the cost. It really isn't bad when you take out the bad stuff from your cart. And next, even if it is more costly, what is the price of a hospital bill for a deadly disease

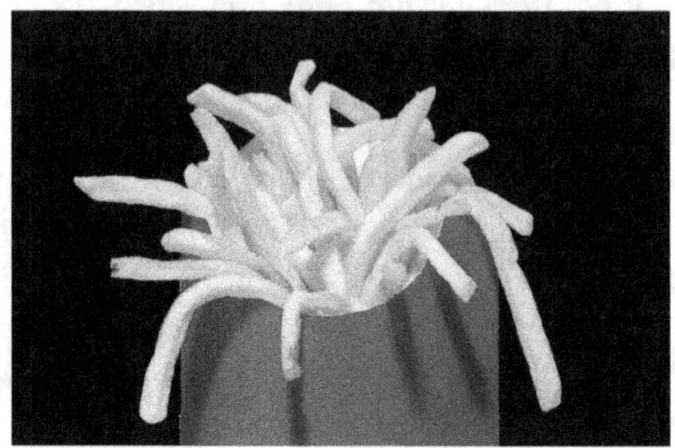

Here is the biggest reason I wanted to write this e-book. Be aware of processed foods. I didn't say be scared or run away, but be aware. I hate the name really, because it could mean so many things. People will say oh my gosh don't eat processed foods. What does processed foods mean? It could be as simple as chopping vegetables and freezing them. Well that doesn't sound scary right? Well that is where other foods could be altered in such a way to be on the scary side. Processed means simply, to alter food from it's original state. When additives, extra sugars, flavorings and preservatives are added, is the scary processed foods we hear about. That is just to name a few things added to make something seem tasty, cheap, and convenient. However we are paying for that convenience with pain, diseases, fatigue, diet pills, and just overall bad health. This is where we really need to eat better and make better decisions.

For starters when sodium is added for preservation you sometimes are looking at twice the recommended daily values for sodium in one meal.

Not only preservatives are added, tons of sugar too. Take a granola bar, this is marketed as a healthy product, which is further from the truth. These bars are loaded with simple sugars which don't satisfy hunger for very long. For one, if that sugar isn't burned off it will turn to fat. But mostly it causes your kidney and liver (your body's detox system) to back up and stress out. These are where pains start to occur. This extra sugar will lead to weight gain and higher blood pressure.

Refined grains is typically a subject that is misunderstood. Let's talk about whole grains VS refined. Put simply, whole grains have had their indigestible hull removed, and refined strips away the bran and germ. With whole grains what is left behind is nutrition, and refined is left with starch and not much else as far as nutrients go.

When reading a nutrition label you will see whole wheat flour or enriched wheat flour, enriched meaning refined. Items that will contain a mix could be bread, pasta, breakfast cereal, crackers, and chips.

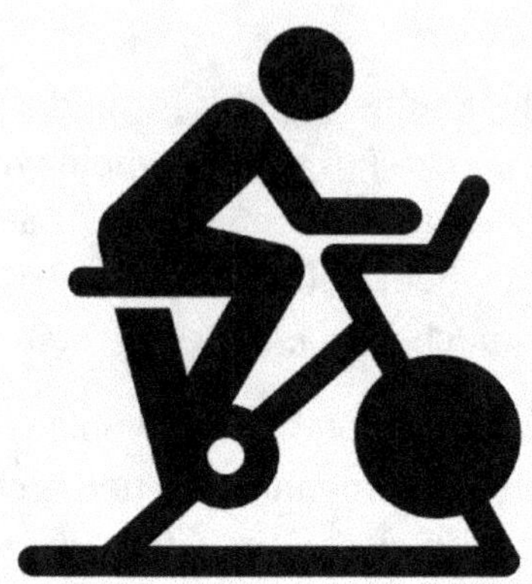

The food you eat really matters for most of your results. However no exercise is going to cause you issues in the long run. One of the big benefits of exercise is long term muscle and bones health.

Overall you will be happier. Changes occur in your brain from exercise that reduce stress and anxiety. It will increase brain sensitivity to serotonin and norepinephrine which fight against depression. A study of both men and women who were exercising regularly were asked to stop and after two weeks experience increasing negative moods.

Yes exercise will help you lose weight. However aside from weight loss, you should look at exercise and weight maintenance. Once you do reach a goal of weight loss, you should either strive for another goal, like adding X amount of pushups, or running 1 mile more or just running faster.

Energy levels will increase with exercise as well. Being fatigued and tired all of the time can be very boring and not very fulfilling in life. When I had a period of time where I had stopped exercising, I would be more tired, slept in and had horrible energy levels. I can't tell you enough how much better I feel, and how good it feels to have energy for the kids.

You will also be reducing your risk of major diseases. To the contrary no exercise, even in the short term can lead to significant increases of belly fat, which is a risk of type 2 diabetes, heart diseases and even early death.

Brain health and memory are improved with better brain function as well because exercise. Basically you are pumping more oxygen to the brain and are stimulating growth of brain cells. Exercise will increase grow your hippocampus (your what?), the part of the brain vital to memory! Exercise also reduces changes in the brain that cause Alzheimer's and schizophrenia.

Are you sleeping poorly? Regular physical activity can help you relax and sleep better. A study shows that around 160 minutes of moderate movement can increase sleep quality 65%. I know after a good workout, or a long day outside, I sleep so good. Sleep is a big part of being healthy as it is. Think of it as a full circle, you work hard to keep your body healthy, your sleep is the time to recover and be ready for the next day.

Exercise also reduces pain, in the past, rest was what doctors prescribed to reduce pain. Now studies have found exercise for those in pain have reduced the pain and increased quality of life. After surgeries they push walking to the patients as quick as they can handle.

If there was one reason to exercise more, this is it, your sex life will improve. Your drive will get a boost, pleasure increases, and so does frequency of night time activities. A group of women in their 40's experienced orgasms more frequently when they included more exercise. Simply by adding regular walks, men who had ED reported a reduction in symptoms by 71%!

The benefits alone should be something to consider if you needed some reasons to increase your physical activity. My favorite of all time I have heard from time to time, is don't you want to look better naked?

Back in the day when I had more time I played flag football in a league with friends. The adrenaline alone is worth the cost to play. We had a great workout each game, and had a lot of fun doing it. I highly recommend exercising with a group. You won't slack off and it's just more fun overall. With the constant sprinting, I need to get in a league again for the workout alone.

If you are stressed out, get a workout in, you will have eliminated or at the worst reduced that stress. There will always be stress in life, even just a little, you will want to find a way to minimize stress the most you can.

The pH scale

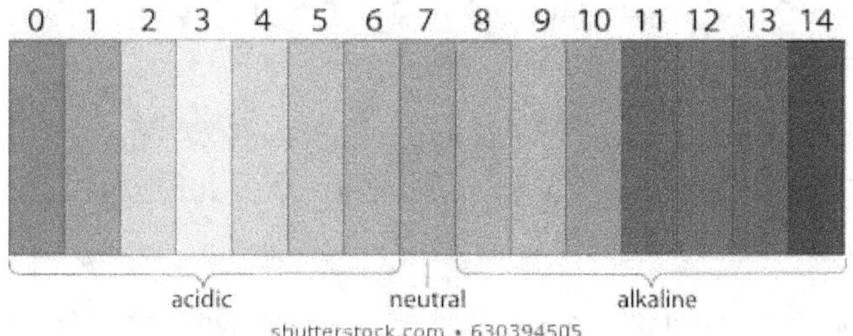

In the best attempt I can, I am leaving science (detailed science that is) out of this book, as I don't want it to be too much science jargon. When I first picked up a couple of health books, the science seemed overwhelming to totally grasp the material.

So what is acid and acidity? From high school chemistry we learned what pH was, and 7 is neutral (neither acidic or alkaline). In short too much acidic foods (no balance) in our system creates an environment where cancer thrives and grows. An alkaline food, and water will help balance out that cup of coffee, and other acid forming foods. Without eating enough alkaline foods our body can regulate our pH anyway and balance for us. Then why worry? Well it only does this to an extent and for so long, eventually it will haunt you.

At the end of the book will be a list of acidic and alkaline foods to help get you on track. Try to make a ratio of 3 to 1 when you eat something like a greasy pizza, cheeseburger, etc. This will help achieve balance. When you eat a complete meal of bad food, don't you feel drained, full and no energy? Balancing this out will make you feel better now, and later too.

Taking this a step further, not all food appears to be acidic. The issue is, the foods can be acid-forming. Which means, a cupcake isn't tart, sour or appears to be acidic. However a cupcake is more acid forming than a lemon. The first time I read this, it blew my mind. I had to look at Google and find a few different sources, but it was true!

Keep in mind not all foods will seem acidic, they will just be acid forming. This is due to a chemical reaction once it hits your enzymes in your mouth.

Other foods to get alkaline forming properties will come from most fruits, vegetables, water, some nuts (not all, check end of book for list). Use the list to help you with balancing out your overall intake. Of course there will be days where you aren't perfect and days you get it right. The key is to balance off those days where you didn't eat too well. Aim for eating mostly alkaline whenever possible, so you won't feel so guilty those other days.

Acidic environments don't just stop with what you eat. This can come from excess stress, unhappiness, and overall negativity. Finding positive things in your life is a must for your body to feel good. There are tons of videos on YouTube about reducing stress in a healthy way.

Take time to keep your environment around you happy, full of positivity and reduce your stress. Wow, this sounds blissful and not easily achievable doesn't it? Try adding a little bit to your life everyday of something positive, just one thing. Next write down something you are grateful for every day.

When you are feeling stressed with work, take a minute to step away and go for a quick walk. Maybe just get a good stretch in, breath in and let it out. Now, slam a glass of water. These simple things can reduce your stress and give you a recharge.

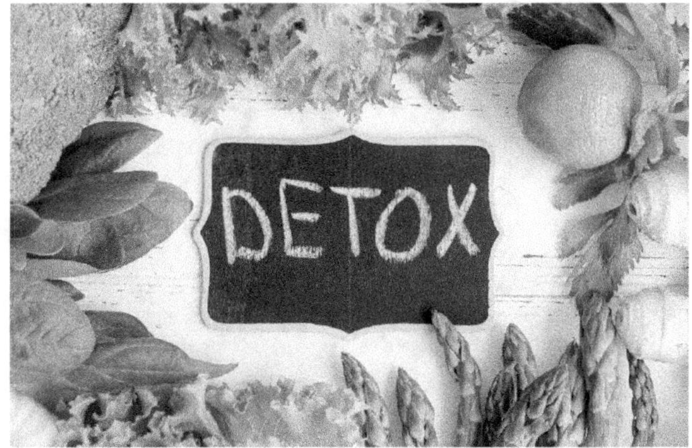

The body has systems in place to help you get rid of toxins, between urination, sweat, your liver and kidneys to name a few. You might have heard of juice cleansers, and other fad diets. They may or may not work, if they do work it is a short-term band aid. What I mean by that is your body needs help and rest with it's detox system. Your body handles toxins for you. That is why I don't do cleansers and such. However like any other system, it can only do so much. You need to help by not over filling the body with toxins and allowing your body to work on it's own.

How can you help your body but not overloading? Watching how many and how much acidic foods, processed foods you are putting in your mouth. By getting the right amount of water and sleep (7-9 hours), and exercising. To really make it easier on your body, eat plenty of greens, veggies, fruits and seeds/nuts. One that might be hard for many, watch your booze intake. Yes, I have a beer at night, but I am not over loading and getting drunk. All of these things will help your body process food better, get rid of toxins and make you feel better over all.

Mindset

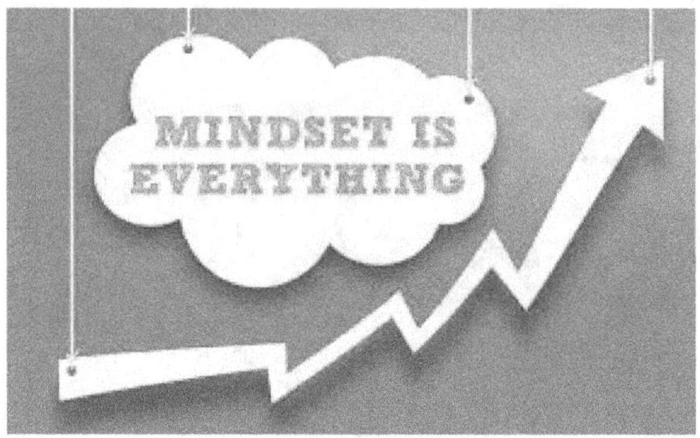

With all of the advice I have given, one secret to bringing this all together is a strong mindset. You will have to have will power. Right now, most will consider having a salad once a week for lunch being healthy. Your ratio of being healthy is way off likely. Once you learn a great variety of healthier foods, your cravings and wants will be more of those foods.

A reason why diets don't work and after the diet is done, most gain the weight back plus more, is they hate what they are eating. If there are certain healthier foods that you don't like, don't eat it! Maybe you add it in to your meal plan here and there, but for the most part, why it's something you don't enjoy. Meals should be enjoyable, not only by taste and fulfilment but also as a break and a breather. If you apply this to your planning for the store or even a garden, you will get more enjoyment out of taking up a healthier lifestyle.

The healthier foods you consume the more you will crave them. As you grow this mindset you will still need to keep your mind sharp. This is for when you want to give into a craving. The problem is, it won't be a small bite to satisfy a craving it will likely be a splurge.

When you are feeling great, take a minute to write down what you did that day and what you ate. The day likely included exercise and healthy eating. This is important to remember on the days you feel like eating a bunch of bad food.

Overall a better mindset will help you in many areas of life. If something bad happens a lot of people can't bounce back right away. Having a stronger mindset prepares you for those moments when life beats you up.

Having a stronger mindset will get you the job at an interview. Think about it, if a person who accepts mediocre results in life is your competition for a job, and you walk in with a great mindset, I think you know who will win the job.

Superfood list

Leafy greens

Goji Berries

Nuts/seeds

Acai

Salmon

Coconut

Tomatoes

Dragonfruit

Garlic

Cauliflower

Broccoli (especially raw)

Tea

Steel Cut Oats

Brown Rice

Lentils

Kiwi

Asparagus

Bananas

Apples

Avacado

Sweet Potato

Berries

Grapes

Most melons

Cherries

Eggs (limit the yolk)

Acid foods to limit (some avoid)

Grains

Sugar

Certain
dairy

Fish

Processed
foods

Fresh meat
and

processed
meat

Soda

French
Fries

White
potatoes

Pizza

Coffee

As long as you limit or avoid more acidic foods you will be fine. I hope you have caught the theme by now, but a balance is what you should strive for. Yes have that slice of pizza, not 5 of them, and wash it down with a salad, glass of water and a bowl of grapes for desert.

Foods that advertised healthy but are not!

Multi-Grain
Bread (not
always, but
mostly not
as healthy
as
advertised)

Energy bars

(artificial
sweeteners
are horrible
for you)

Labeled
Sugar Free

Fat free or
low fat

(instead of
fat, sugar is
replaced to
enhance
flavor)

Flavored
Oatmeal

Dried fruit

Baked chips
(yes better,
not great)

Yogurt
covered
raisins

Pita chips

Sports
drinks

Diet Soda

Bottom line, watch for what ingredients are in the foods you are buying, what did they pump in there to enhance shelf life? With food colorings, preservatives, artificial sweeteners, added sugars, healthier foods are turned into bad foods just like that.

Food suggestions

The following vitamins and minerals are just suggestions, there are more possibilities of course. As preached thus far in this book, it is about balance. Have fun with seeking a balance from these foods and don't be afraid to try something new!

<u>Minerals</u>

Protein – almonds, beans, chickpeas, eggs, kale, lentils, pumpkin seeds, quinoa, seaweed, sunflower seeds, & tempeh

Good fats – almonds/almond butter, avocados, chia seed, coconut oil, cold pressed extra virgin oil, freshly ground flax seed, sacha inchi oil, walnuts

Fats are good as long as we get the right ones. Your body doesn't produce essential fatty acids, so we need to provide them.

Minerals – alfalfa sprouts, broccoli, cabbage, garlic, hazelnuts, kale, oats

Around 4% of our body mass is made of minerals, it is important to keep these available in the body.

Calcium – apricots, brussels sprouts, butternut squash, cabbages, chard, figs, kelp, pistachios, plum, sesame seeds, spinach, turnips

Calcium contributes to bone and teeth health. It also a main buffer when the body is in acidosis.

Magnesium – Asparagus, avocado, bananas, beet greens, brazil nuts, brown rice, cashews, kiwis, peas, prunes, squash

Helps with insulin, hormone, and fat metabolism regulation

Potassium – acorn squash, broccoli, cabbage, carrots, cherries, currant, kiwi, mushrooms, peanuts, sweat potato

Needed for fluid and electrolyte balance. This directly effects blood pressure and pH balance. Responsible for communication between nerve and muscle.

Iron – coconuts, legumes, macadamia nuts, oats, quinoa, raisins, sesame seeds, sun-dried tomatoes, swiss chard, watercress

Required for vital biological function

Copper – apricots, cashews, coconut, hazelnuts, kale, peaches, pecans, portobello mushrooms, shiitake mushrooms, walnuts

Regulates cholesterol, fights infections and helps tissue repair

Zinc – asparagus, green peas, lemongrass, Napa cabbage, oats, pecans, prunes, pumpkin seeds, shiitake mushrooms, spinach

Key element in metabolism of RNA and DNA.

Phosphorus – alfalfa sprouts, avocados, broccoli, celery, chia seeds, kiwi fruit, pistachios, watercress, wild rice, zucchini

The basic structure of DNA/RNA is made up of phosphorus.

Manganese – blueberries, chilies, collared greens, currant, eggplant, garlic, grapes, leeks, pumpkin seeds, raspberries

Provides proper brain, bone, and liver health.

Selenium – asparagus, brazil nuts, broccoli, brussels sprouts, coconut, garlic, grapefruit, mushrooms, spinach, sunflower seeds

Essential for heart, blood and thyroid health.

Vitamins

Vitamin A – Avocado, bell peppers, cantaloupe, carrots, chili peppers, collard greens, mangoes, spinach, sweet potatoes

Essential for proper vision, skin, antioxidant function, and immune system maintenance.

Vitamin B – brown rice, cabbage, legumes, yogurt, nuts, seeds, quinoa, wild mushrooms

Vitamin B plays a key role in cell function and biological functions. Limitless benefits of optimal health.

Vitamin C- bok choy, broccoli, brussels sprouts, citrus fruits, kiwi, papaya, peppers, pineapple, raspberries, strawberries

Responsible for key enzymatic reactions involved in collagen formation. Has roles in maintaining immune, antihistamine, antioxidant

Vitamin D – mushrooms (specifically chanterelle, oyster, portobello, shiitake and cremini).

Vital for key biological functions such as calcium and phosphate gut uptake, bone and neuromuscular health, immune health and many others. This is one of those vitamins especially if you live in colder states for the winter (less sun), you might want to take a vitamin d supplement.

Vitamin E – almonds, avocados, brazil nuts, chia, cod-liver oil, cold-pressed extra virgin olive oil, freshly ground flax seed, peanut butter, quinoa, sunflower seeds, walnuts

Helps antioxidant process in the body, tissue repair, neurological functions and more.

Vitamin K – basil, beet greens, bok choy, broccoli, brussels sprouts, kale, pumpkin seeds, spinach, turnips

Important for blood clotting and bone and cardio health.

As mentioned before listing off the different suggestions don't be limited to this list. And be sure to strike a balance. After all that is what is the spice of life, more balance right?

Here are some more suggestions for different functions.

Fiber – all whole veggies and fruits, apples, beans, chia seeds, chickpeas, coconut, oats, pumpkin seeds, quinoa, walnuts

Fiber assists digestive tract to do its job properly.

Detoxify – all fruits and veggies, berries, chillies, fermented foods like kefir, sauerkraut, garlic, greens, herbs, raw apple cider vinegar, seaweed, sprouts, turmeric

All of these foods help rid the body of toxins.

Antioxidants – artichoke hearts, avocado, beans, berries, oregano, pecans, pomegranates, prunes, quinoa, spices like cloves, cumin, curry, cinnamon, and vanilla.

These foods will counteract the harmful oxidation caused by free radicals.

Anti-inflammatory – alliums (onion, garlic, & leeks), olive oil, yogurt, flaxseed, ginger, green tea, hazel nuts, macadamia nuts, rosemary, seaweed

Stress and dehydration create chronic inflammation that can lead to chronic diseases. These foods assist the body in regulating inflammation and nourishing the damaged areas.

Prebiotics – agave, alliums, apples, asparagus, bananas, cruciferous vegetables like cabbage and broccoli, greens, oats, papaya, quinoa, walnuts

These foods create favorable conditions for the healthy microbes our bodies need.

Probiotics – apple cider vinegar, fermented foods such as sauerkraut, kimchi, kombucha, miso, olives, kefir, yogurt, tempeh

Fermentation is an ancient process that gives food a longer shelf life. The process also forms beneficial flora into the digestive system where we need them.

Immune system support – aloe vera, echinacea, garlic, ginger, goldenseal, mushrooms, onion, organic local honey, oxygen and alkaline foods

Certain foods supply us with essential nutrients and important nonessential molecules that play roles in activating and regulating our body's defense system.

Brain support – blueberries, nuts, coconut oil, cod-liver oil, green tea, quinoa, rosemary

The brain is the most metabolically active part of your body and most important too. It requires lots of nutrition to function properly.

Good for your blood – alliums, beets, chia seeds, chili peppers, cilantro, citrus, coconut water, parsley, pomegranates, seaweed

Stress – chamomile, ginseng, licorice root, passionflower, raw nuts, skullcap, valerian

Energy – apple cider vinegar, chili peppers, ginseng, green tea, kimchi, raw local honey, quinoa, reishi mushrooms, sprouts, yerba mate

Joints – avocado, black pepper, chili peppers, coconut oil, cod-liver oil, olive oil, ginger, nuts, pineapple, turmeric

Sex – avocado, cacao, fenugreek seeds, garlic, ginseng, pumpkin seeds, quinoa, raw local honey

Skin – almonds, avocado, berries, nuts, citrus, coconut oil, cod-liver oil, pumpkin seeds, quinoa, sesame oil

Eyes – avocado, bilberries, eyebright, fennel, grape seeds, greens, green tea, milk thistle, saffron, tomatoes

Muscles – almonds, nuts, chia seeds, eggs, garlic, greens, pumpkin seeds, quinoa

Anti-cancer foods – alliums, leafy greens, berries, fermented foods, nuts, quinoa, spices, sweet potatoes, tea

Healthy sweeteners – agave syrup, blackstrap molasses, coconut sugar, date sugar, honey, lo han guo, maple syrup, stevia, yacon syrup

I'll say it again, these suggestions shouldn't be your limit. I mostly want to get you started is all. Making small changes and a shift in mindset was what helped me start to feel healthier and lose more and more weight.

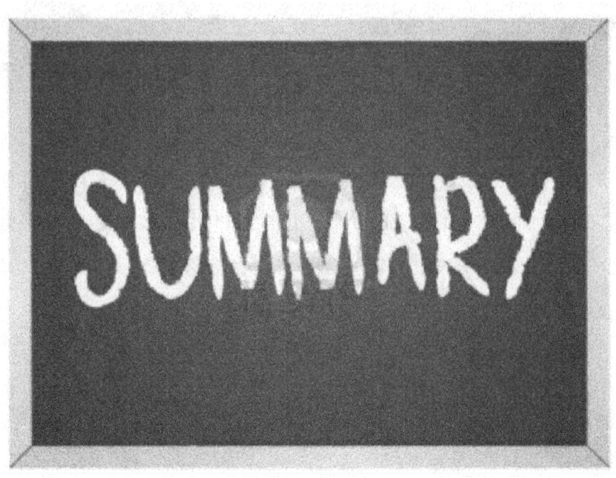

As with anything in life you need to strike a balance. If you know you haven't been exercising lately, watch your food intake and try to cut something out as you know you won't burn it off (or just increase your exercise). Look at sugar, we need sugar, but we need to limit and watch our intake of sugar especially.

Be sure to drink plenty of water and get exercise. When days are bad, stressed, or just short on time, try to at least sneak in some push ups, leg lifts or crunches at the minimum. When my family was going through a move and trying to find houses during COVID-19, we were short on time and high on stress. Being sure to get my pushups in, it made me feel better and kept me on track. Even with all the chaos, I was still eating better than the year before.

There will be days when you want to just eat a large pizza by yourself, if you are on a trend of losing weight try to hold back. Have a slice or two and enjoy it, but wash it down with some salad and water. I say this, as you have to make those tougher choices and not give in. If you give in now, you will again. I get it your busy, and it's so much easier to order a pizza. Keep your mindset strong and ready to fight these cravings.

Remember the old mentality, oh it's ok enjoy the burger now and then. Well the folks who usually told me that also ate like crap on other days as well. It should be more on the veggies and foods to make you feel good. Those conversations need to be more common. Have conversations with like minded people on the subject too.

Having a like minded group with similar goals will help keep you going. A group can usually offer advice when needed. Even better, a group of people with different ideas can all help each other way more than this book. This book is meant to get you started.

Maybe you need a reason why? Why do you want more energy, to feel better, look better, and live longer? Is it for your spouse? Your kids? Find a reason that will drive you. Just a goal to lose 5lbs will run out of steam eventually. Have a strong "why", will take you further and keep this lifestyle alive.

When you feel like quitting, having a strong why will keep you going. The reason behind the why is a huge driver for many success stories in human history. Your why will motivate you, and push you beyond your limits. Your body was designed to slow down once you were going full steam. The reason is, your body thinks it needs to save energy for later. That is part from evolution when food was scarce, this isn't the case now.

If you feel like you have pain, or just don't love your body now, why accept anything less. We have one life on this planet, make the most out of it comfortably. There is no reason to wake up everyday grumpy, full of hate and pains.

Be better, eat better, feel better.

P.S. For Smokers

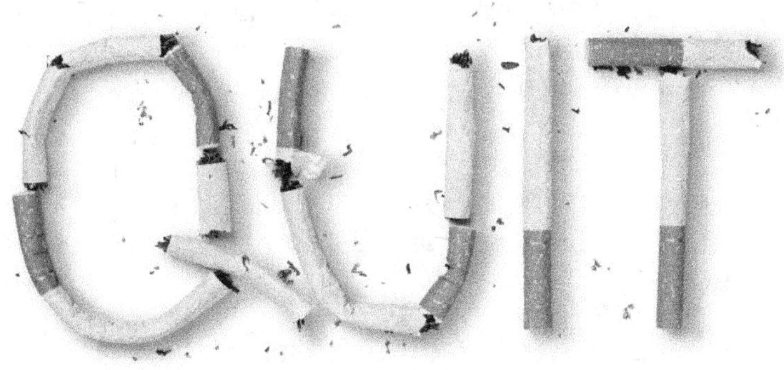

As a former smoker myself, one thing that happened to me was gain weight right away. I didn't care at the time as I knew my snacking was suppressing my cravings. I didn't care as I knew the cravings for a cig would go away and I would be healthier. That all might be true, I just wish I was snacking on something different. If I were to do that now, I would have had sliced peppers to eat as I worked, apples, nuts, and stuff like that.

Either way, quitting smoking was a great achievement for me and I recommend you trying as well. There is nothing healthy about it.

New Discoveries

It has been so awesome since I first released the original version of the e-book. It has meant so much to me to hear how so many have changed ways of their eating and how much better they feel. Success stories I receive have been amazing.

I have a few short stories to share with you below on some of the stories I have got so far, and I hope this gives you more motivation!

The stories go beyond health and fitness, I chose the ones who also had a life changing experience outside of better eating and exercise. These all hit me the same way, as I got better at my sales job because I had more energy and just felt better about life and it translated to my work life as well. I was so happy to see this happened to others as well.

Christine 38, Colorado. Since I read this book not only have, I lost weight I feel great too. Every day I wanted to quit my job and do something better, and finally I did. Now I feel great about my job, and everyday life.

Matt 29, California. As a military veteran myself I related too closely when you said you gained weight right after you got out. I did the same, except I kept going and gained over 115 pounds. Since reading your book I have been exercising, eating better and slowly chopping off the pounds. I even went on my first date in years.

Gary 46 Nevada. I have been working in an office since college and have not exercised in years. This book was suggested by a friend and I dove right in. After just one month of changing what I eat, and minimal exercise (I'm getting there), I feel amazing now. Going out for walks used to sound boring and a waste of time, now I crave it.